Leptin Reset!

14 Days to Resetting Your Leptin and Turning Your Body Into a Fat-Burning Machine

Sara Givens

DEDICATION

To Mr. Rice, my favorite gym teacher who always encouraged me to do one more rep.

CONTENTS

Introduction: The Weight Loss Dilemma

Let me ask you a simple question. How long have you struggled to lose weight? Probably all your life, right? And how many times have you slashed your calories and did so much cardio that you felt like your legs were going to fall off, only to have all the weight come right back again when you stopped? Frustrating doesn't even begin to describe how you really feel, does it?

But don't give up just yet--not until you read this. I know you want to blame yourself; but the truth is, it really is not your fault.

Over the past 40 years, there's been a lot of research into food, dieting, disease, and metabolism. Most of the scientific findings fly in the face of 'conventional' food wisdom, and many of those researchers have been labeled 'radicals' and the results of their studies buried under a barrage of bad press. The official line still calls for a diet based on eating mostly carbohydrates, severely limiting fats, increasing exercise, and counting calories.

While we've been following that official advice from the 'experts', the rates of obesity, diabetes, cardiovascular disease, cancer, and autoimmune diseases have dramatically and steadily risen. They say that this new generation is the first in history to face the likelihood of not living as long as their parents did, or as healthily. It's predicted that by 2030, almost 80% of the population will be diabetic or pre-diabetic. Like many of us, you may have found out personally that it just doesn't work, and you may have begun to doubt 'conventional wisdom' and the 'official line'.

If you're part of the growing 'been there, done that ... and the tee shirt don't fit no more' group, then you are in good company. Isn't it time you learned how your body really functions, based on valid modern scientific studies from the world's top scientific and medical research labs?

Don't worry, you don't need a Ph.D. in biology to understand the basics of how your metabolism works. Once you understand just a few simple facts about your hormones, you'll hold the key to controlling not just your weight, but also your sleep, your moods, your overall health, and your longevity.

One hormone in particular that holds the key to fat loss is called leptin. Leptin is a hormone that decreases appetite while simultaneously increasing your metabolism. If you think that sounds pretty important, you would be right. Hormones are the chemical messengers for your brain, and if those messages can't be read properly, things won't work the way they should. Just as insulin resistance leads to diabetes, leptin resistance leads to obesity and a host of other health problems. If you want to lose weight and keep it off, you need to understand leptin.

In this book, you'll discover how hormones, in general, control every aspect of your life and how leptin, in particular, functions to promote and maintain a healthy body and healthy weight. What's more, you'll learn how what you eat affects your hormones, why and how you can become 'resistant' to these chemical messages, and exactly what you can do to turn things around.

Dr. Barry Sears, a leading authority on controlling hormones through diet, said in his 1995 book *The Zone,* 'food is the most powerful drug you will ever encounter' (p. 27). It's time to learn how to put food to work *for* you instead of *against* you. Simple changes in your diet and lifestyle can reset your leptin sensitivity, and make your body return to functioning the way nature intended. It's time to try what works. If you're ready for that, read on!

Chapter I: Your Hormones and Metabolism

Much of what we've been taught about metabolism is incorrect. The 'eat less and exercise more' versions of diets are dinosaurs that ignore the current known facts about how our bodies actually function. Dietary recommendations are completely out-of-date, and in many instances they simply make our problems worse. The media and the Internet bury us with information on the latest diet craze, but they don't tell us what we really need to know ... and we get heavier, sicker, and more worn out, week by week and year by year.

The calories in theory is an over simplification of the process and not the way your body really uses energy. What happens is much more complex, and it's mostly controlled by your hormones.

Most people are only aware of a few hormones that regulate the functioning of their bodies on a daily basis --- testosterone, estrogen, insulin, and adrenaline, for instance. They've gotten a lot of press. But with our current weight crisis, how many metabolic hormones have you heard about? Precious few, most likely.

Sorry to have to go into geek mode on you but it's important you understand some hormone basics as they are related to leptin and fat loss.

In 1902, two British physiologists identified the first hormones and created the word 'hormone'. Taken from the Greek, 'hormone' means 'that which sets in motion'. That's what hormones do; they are the catalysts for most processes, feelings, and reactions in our bodies. More than 100 hormones have now been identified, and they affect the activity of every cell in our body.

Recent studies have even shown that certain hormones can activate receptors in the nucleus of cells and bind themselves to individual genes in the DNA, activating certain genetic components and deactivating others. Hormones do indeed form an intricate network of chemical messages circulating through your body.

Hormones are produced primarily by the endocrine system of glands, but other organs and tissue produce them as well. Ultimately, they affect mental acuity, physical growth, reproduction, digestion, metabolism, heart rate, blood pressure, mood, sleep quality, and our 'fight-or-flight' responses. Dr. Barry Sears, a leading biochemist studying hormones, put it very succinctly when he said 'to control your hormones is to control your life'.

So what controls and directs your hormones? You do.

That's right ... you control them through the food you eat, the way you handle stress, and how much you work with your biology instead of against it.

There are several major hormones that work to maintain, regulate, and distribute the available energy to the various functions your body needs to carry out. Many of these actions are beyond your control, such as the energy needed for breathing, brain function, and blood circulation. These functions form your basal metabolism, the energy your body requires to continue living. Beyond that, some energy will be allotted for both cellular and general body repair. This is why you feel tired and sleep more when you're sick or badly injured. Your system is using extra energy to heal and fight disease, and it has decreased the amount available for 'awake' functions.

Your body also maintains stores of energy to protect itself from a lack of food in the future. Some of that is tucked away in your large muscles, but the majority of the extra is stashed in the body's pantry: fat cells. Since you only need a certain amount for normal body functioning, if you over-consume energy (that is, calories), your system will save all the extra as fat.

Believe it or not, some scientists actually consider some types of body fat to be an organ of the body. There are two kinds of fat, white and brown. White fat is stored energy that we see as 'love handles' and a 'spare tire'. If we lack food for a prolonged period, it will be used to maintain all the workings of our system.

Brown fat is the one you don't hear much about. It's the 'good' fat, if you want to think of it that way, because brown fat actually burns calories all the time. Athletes, young people, and thin people have a good amount of brown fat working for them.

Another hormone called ghrelin produces feelings of hunger, signaling your body to seek food.

But before you even chew or swallow that food, your taste buds will send out a message that food is in your mouth, triggering the release of insulin. Insulin works to control the amount of glucose, or blood sugar, keeping it within acceptable levels.

The digestive hormones trigger the release of enzymes to break down the food into nutrients and energy. Glucagon controls the storage of energy in muscle tissue, and leptin signals when you've had enough, so you won't overeat and upset the balance.

Adding to the intricacy of this whole process is the timing of hormone release. Some are released overnight, some only in the day. Some hormones will only be produced when certain other conditions exist, such as deep REM sleep between midnight and 2 a.m. Many hormones affect the production or quantity of other hormones, so the correct balance needs to be maintained.

Since most of them are affected by the fuel we give our bodies, it's important to understand how hormones work ... and what you can do to keep them working properly. Many people with weight or health issues will not see any long-term improvement or success until they reset and regulate their hormones.

The Ship's Captain of Fat Loss

One of the most important hormones for achieving and maintaining a healthy body weight and a normal metabolism appears to be leptin. When leptin signals you to stop eating, it's because it is the ultimate controller of energy consumption. It's in charge of the overall plan for energy usage and sends out messages that affect the other metabolic hormones telling them what to do.

Just as the captain of a ship is ultimately responsible for everything from food to cargo to safety, leptin is the body's captain as far as metabolism goes. It sets and oversees the entire energy plan, and the other hormones are responsible for implementing it. So anything that affects your leptin levels can throw your entire metabolism out of whack, and correcting these problems can return your metabolism to its ideal state. When your metabolism is functioning properly, you'll lose excess body fat rather easily and keep it off as you resolve and prevent many health problems.

Chapter II: Understanding Leptin Resistance

Fat-storage is hard-wired into our genetic code, and unfortunately we can't change it. We are genetically pre-disposed by thousands of years of existence toward the 'feast-or-famine' framework, and our bodies are ever alert to possible starvation. We have to learn to work with it, and to control or regulate the hormonal messages that signal a lack of food. When you follow a conventional diet and restrict calories, your brain says "Whoa! Starvation alert!' and switches into high gear as far as storing fat goes.

Your overall metabolism is slowed down to allow this to happen, and weight loss becomes very difficult. A slower metabolism also makes us feel lazier and less inclined to exercise, so we won't use as much energy. If you manage to lose weight anyway, your system is just waiting for food to become plentiful again so it can replenish its stores, and the weight is regained. So you try a different diet, with the same end result. This is called yo-yo dieting.

Over-exposure to something decreases our sensitivity to it, and we tolerate it more. It becomes more acceptable to us. That's one of the objections to violent computer games and films. If you use a lot of salt on your food, you don't taste it as much. Go totally off all salt for a few weeks, and you'll find the same amount to be way too much, making the food almost inedible. You've reset your salt sensitivity.

The same thing happens with natural substances produced by our bodies. Diabetes is the result of the system becoming desensitized to insulin. It stops 'reading' the chemical message that insulin delivers and therefore it doesn't react by controlling blood sugar. This is known as insulin resistance, that is, the body has become resistant to using insulin properly. The increased levels of insulin no longer trigger the series of processes in the way they should. The same thing happens with leptin. An overabundance of leptin over time can make your system lose its sensitivity to it. In effect, it stops listening. Since leptin is the controller of metabolism, leptin resistance means bad things for your body.

The question, of course, is why you would have 'too much' leptin in the first place. There are many factors that play into the answer to this question, so let's look at some of them. The easiest one is that leptin is produced by fat cells, so the more fat you carry, the higher your leptin levels. Yep, and some of you have always jumped ahead and seen the Catch-22 here! As you gain weight, you produce more leptin and your body doesn't listen to it as much. The messages have become too constant, and desensitization occurs. The extra fat that's gained produces an even higher level in your blood. You're quickly in leptin overload. It's a vicious cycle. Once your body stops listening to its leptin, it believes it's in 'starvation' mode and no diet in the world will take the weight off and keep it off. The captain of the metabolic ship is being ignored. You need to re-sensitize your system to leptin and bring your levels under control to lose weight.

While you can't wave a magic wand to reduce the amount of body fat you carry, and therefore the amount of leptin you produce, there are a number of other factors that contribute to leptin resistance. It's through those other avenues that you can reset your leptin receptors so that they'll read your leptin levels correctly. In other words, you can't necessarily change your leptin levels without reducing body fat, but you can get your brain to start interpreting the messages correctly once again. Once the levels are being 'listened to' properly, your metabolism will react accordingly, and you'll be able to lose weight without cravings or hunger.

One factor in resetting your leptin is to let your metabolism rest naturally overnight on a regular basis. Most of your leptin is produced during the last four hours of sleep. There are two main things involved with that process. First, you need to stop eating. Your system needs time to finish the digestion process before it can settle into making its metabolic plans for the next day. Snacking in the evening seriously interferes with that process, causing a release of insulin that re-stimulates the metabolism. There's not enough time between a bedtime snack at 10 p.m. and getting up at 6 a.m. for the whole process to work through. You need at least eleven hours in between, so you'll need to stop eating three to four hours before bedtime to help your body begin to read leptin correctly again.

It can seem very challenging to work this into your daily schedule. Modern work schedules have shifted 'normal' dinnertime to later in the evening. Fifty years ago, most people had dinner between 5 and 6 p.m., which allowed that 11+ hours before breakfast in the morning. Our later evening meals have interfered with our metabolic function, and it's no coincidence that the 'fattening' of the population began at the same time that dinnertime started getting later and later. If you add on munching in front of the TV after that evening meal, you've further messed with the system.

Simply not going to bed until at least three hours after finishing dinner isn't a real solution either. Unless your morning schedule is extremely flexible, you'll be cutting into your sleep time --- and good sleep is another factor in resetting your leptin. Research studies in the late 1990's showed a very clear link between sleep deprivation and weight gain. I'm not just talking about getting by on five hours a night here! A normal adult needs seven to nine hours of quality sleep every night or you become 'sleep deprived'. For optimal health and function, most people need two sleep cycles a night, with a cycle varying from three-and-a-half to four-and-a-half hours, depending on the individual. As you know, when you are deep asleep your system slows down --- heart rate, breathing, the works. The energy saved by this slow-down is used for repair, maintenance, and general assessment of the whole system. Part of that assessment is your leptin levels, which are used to determine your metabolic rate for the following day and the need, or lack thereof, to store fat.

It's not just the quantity of sleep that matters; it's the quality as well. A night spent tossing and turning interferes with the sleep cycles, and so it prevents our body from taking care of necessary jobs. The reason it's hard to wake up and think clearly after the alarm jolts you out of a dream is because your system has had to drop what it was doing during that sleep cycle, and it suddenly has to resume its 'day job'. That means that some very important biological tasks, many on the cellular level, are left unfinished. We can handle it on an occasional basis; but like any other intricate system, constant neglect of routine maintenance inevitably leads to trouble.

Many things can adversely affect your sleep. Establishing and keeping both a bedtime routine and a schedule can help improve your ability to fall asleep as well as your sleep quality. So can setting up a good sleep environment that's dark and quiet. Lowering the overall amount of light during the evening can encourage our natural inclination to sleep when it's dark, and turning off the electronics at least an hour before bed has the same effect. If you have trouble sleeping, do some online research into ways that you can improve the quality, quantity, and regularity of your sleep. It's important not only for weight loss but also for all other aspects of your health and happiness.

To reset your leptin, you also need to clean up the food you eat. Most food additives are known to interfere with hormones in various ways, and they confuse leptin receptors in particular. Certain additives are known to block leptin from crossing the blood-brain barrier and delivering its message. Artificial sweeteners are notorious for messing up your body's messaging system. They trigger insulin production, which in turn sets off storing energy as fat, and they also appear to interfere with the action of leptin receptors, preventing your brain from getting the message that you are full and already have enough fat in storage.

Dr. Joseph Mercola, a leading researcher and writer on health issues, sums up the process as follows: "In a nutshell, when you eat something sweet, your brain releases dopamine, which supplies you with a jolt of pleasure. Your brain's reward center is activated. The appetite-regulating hormone leptin is also released, which eventually informs your brain that you are 'full' once a certain amount of calories have been ingested.

In contrast, when you consume something sweet but non-caloric (i.e. an artificial sweetener), your brain's pleasure pathway is still activated by the sweet taste, but there's nothing to **de**activate it, since your body is still waiting for the calories." ("The Aspartame End Game...and What's Next". 4/16/2014. articles.mercola.com)

Your body will continue to signal you to eat until it gets the calories it was promised. Hello, snacking!

The consumer advocacy group US Right to Know has filed a citizen petition to the FDA, asking for investigation of any food labeled 'diet' which contains artificial sweeteners. Gary Ruskin, executive director of that organization, said, "We have asked the FTC and the FDA to shut down what appears to be a consumer fraud." In their letter to the FDA, RTK stated "their use of the term 'diet' in advertising for these products appears to be deceptive ... because scientific evidence suggests artificial sweeteners contribute to weight gain, not weight loss ..." (as quoted in "Could This Headache Causing Neurotoxin Be on Its Way Out?" 5/15/2015. http://articles.mercola.com).

Breaking leptin resistance is dependent on eating natural, real food, without additives, pesticides, added hormones, or processing. These all place stress on your system, and the quantity of them in our food supply has dramatically increased over the past 25 years. This stress is manifested as inflammation, which is now believed to be a major contributor to the development of many serious diseases. This inflammation is on the interior of the body, around organs, blood vessels, intestines, and individual cells throughout every system. It's a reaction to things that are eaten but don't register as 'food'. Some of these substances are even stored away in our fat cells, since the human body doesn't know what else to do with them.

High fructose corn syrup is one that I'm sure you've read about. It's all over the health news, isn't it? Fructose is a form of sugar found naturally in fruit. For most of human history, summer was 'feast' and winter was 'famine'. Our systems needed to store fat to see us through the winter. We therefore developed a great survival ability to store the fructose from summer's bounty as fat, and to later use that stored energy to supplement winter's meager food supply. It worked great until the growth of agriculture, when we no longer had to rely on so much stored fat for surviving the winter. Once food became adequate year-round, we lost our need to stockpile fat. However, biologically we continue to be great at storing fructose!

We don't actually need very much fructose. The liver metabolizes it, and if needed, it's turned into glycogen and stored. Most people already have enough glycogen, however, so the liver converts this fructose into fats called triglycerides, a major risk factor for heart disease. When your liver has as much of these fats as it can hold (fatty liver is a health problem of its own), the triglycerides are leaked out into your blood stream. If you've had a cholesterol test done, it measured not only HDL and LDL, but also triglycerides. Lots of people have elevated levels of triglycerides, and it's because of fructose, not dietary fat.

Fructose has yet another bad effect on us --- it doesn't satisfy. In a study done at the Yale University School of Medicine and published in the *Journal of the American Medical Association* in 2013, it was found that fructose doesn't promote a feeling of fullness like other sugars do. Another study showed that fructose doesn't lower the level of ghrelin, the hormone that stimulates your feeling of hunger. The end result is that consuming fructose doesn't satisfy your hunger, so you eat more.

Now think about the effect of all the high-fructose corn syrup that's currently being added to processed foods under various names. We excel at storing it as fat, not burning it for energy. It raises triglycerides, contributing to heart disease, and it doesn't fill you up so you still feel hungry. None of this is good for your health or your weight. In fact, it's working *against* your efforts to lose weight!

You may not be aware that sugar, regular table sugar (sucrose), is 50% fructose. Therefore, all foods containing sugar are working against you in several ways. Unfortunately, the sugars in processed foods can be be listed under about 60 different names, making it very difficult to tell how much sugar you're actually consuming. Sadly, even many 'weight loss' foods contain sugar and/or artificial sweeteners, under one name or another, which means that these foods are urging your body to gain weight, not lose it.

Other additives and ingredients in processed foods have the same type of effects on our systems, and I won't detail all of them here. To lower your leptin resistance, you need to return to eating 'real' food, food that hasn't been processed. That said, you don't need to make everything from scratch, either.

What you need to learn to do is to read food labels. Reading labels takes some practice, but learning the common names for added sugar is a good place to start. Sugar gets added to all sorts of things, including toothpaste! If it sounds processed (like 'partially hydrogenated'), stay away from it. Some prepared items will surprise you, pleasantly. Let me give you an example.

I have a jar of unsweetened applesauce in my pantry, from a major national food company. It contains apples, water, and ascorbic acid. That's the entire ingredient list, just as it should be. [If you're wondering, ascorbic acid keeps the apples from turning dark brown, and home cooks often use citric acid (lemon juice) for the same purpose.] So you don't need to make your own applesauce or pasta or jam, you just need to find the right brand.

Start by checking out the things in your pantry. Read the labels on the things you use often. That will point you toward the good brands, like my applesauce, that you want to continue buying, and you'll learn the not-so-good ones, like some instant mashed potatoes I bought that have four kinds of sugar in them. Really! You'll shop slower when you first start weeding out the overly-processed foods. Once you find a good brand, your grocery shopping will speed right back up. Enlist the help of your children and spouse to do the label reading in the pantry and on the first couple of shopping trips. Kids are great at this, and they can become little tyrants about it, too. If you don't find what you're looking for in the regular aisles, try the organic section. Removing these unnatural additions from your food is key in losing weight, reclaiming your health, and resetting your leptin levels.

Not consuming enough fiber and protein has also been linked to leptin resistance, as has the overconsumption of carbohydrates. Readjusting your daily percentages of these macronutrients can help reset your sensitivity to leptin and get your metabolism back on track. A lack of regular exercise also contributes to leptin resistance. It's not the intensity of the exercise but the consistency in doing it that helps your metabolic functions return to normal. A regular walk around the block after dinner can get you away from food and provide much needed exercise.

As you can see, there are many things affecting the ability of leptin to regulate your metabolism. The leptin reset diet will address all these issues, lowering your resistance to leptin and letting your entire system return to functioning as it was meant to. You will lose weight and begin to see a number of other related improvements in your overall health and performance.

Chapter III: Signs and Symptoms of Leptin Resistance

How do you know if you're leptin resistant? If you're struggling with your weight or any chronic health issues, it's likely that your leptin levels are not registering with your brain. Leptin is involved with the proper functioning of so many systems in the body that any list of symptoms appears long. Let's divide them into groups for clarity.

Weight Issues

Being *overweight* automatically raises your leptin levels since it is produced by fat cells. If you have made 'good faith' efforts to lose weight without much success, you are probably leptin resistant. If you have regained weight following successful dieting, or only lose a small amount (5-10 lbs.) no matter what you do, your metabolism is not responding to your leptin. Although it's not discussed as often, being chronically *underweight* is also a sign of leptin malfunction. Those low levels of leptin should be telling the body to eat more, but they're not. There is currently research in progress to verify whether leptin resistance plays a physical part in anorexia.

Leptin resistance typically results in abdominal fat, the classic apple shape that is now known to be a risk factor in many serious diseases. A 'pooch', 'muffin top', or 'beer belly' is a good indicator of leptin resistance.

Appetite

Unless you're a growing teenager, your appetite should prompt you to eat about 1600 to 2000 calories a day. That's for a normal adult with normal activity levels. If this is not enough to satisfy your hunger, then your leptin is not controlling your system the way it should. A *big appetite* for your age and activity level is a sure sign of leptin resistance. Eating overly large meals before you register 'I'm full' is another symptom. *Overeating* is a sign that there's major interference in the messages being exchanged between your stomach and your brain.

Snacking and Cravings

Snacking can just be a bad habit, but it can also be a sign that your brain has decided you need to seek food. If you've had an adequate meal, you shouldn't feel any need to nibble every few hours, so your brain is not getting the correct information from your leptin.

Cravings are similar to snacking. If you're used to eating a highly processed high-carb diet, you may feel cravings for carbs, especially in the evenings. Cravings are often misinterpreted as a biological need for a particular food. If you're craving 'salty crunchy', it has very little to do with salt. It's the carbs in the potato chips, pretzels, or popcorn that your system is wanting, so it can turn them into fat and raise your leptin levels. It's the same if you're craving fruit, except fructose and carbs is the objective. Cravings are a symptom of leptin malfunction.

Stress and Mood Swings

Stress produces a hormone called cortisol, which interferes with your metabolism in two ways. First it prevents your brain from reading leptin levels properly and, second, cortisol interferes with your sleep. As discussed earlier, much of the metabolic planning for your system is done during sleep, including leptin production. Bad sleep equals bad metabolic function. The correlation between poor sleep and weight gain was discovered back in the 1980's, but it's taken longer to pin down the hormones responsible.

Chronic stress combined with poor quality sleep results in hormone imbalances that directly affect mood. These imbalances produce *mood swings* and frequent *irritability,* and ultimately point to leptin issues. De-stressing on a regular basis is important to lower leptin resistance. Regular exercise helps with this, as does learning to deal with stress better through meditation or hobbies.

Fatigue and Insomnia
Although these symptoms may have many causes, frequent fatigue and/or insomnia affect your body's ability to take care of the metabolic assessment and allocation that takes place in deep sleep. This results in overall hormone difficulties, but since leptin is the master hormone for metabolism, these problems can produce sluggish or non-reactions from leptin receptors.

Many food additives, as well as sugar, are known to interfere with deep sleep, promoting not only insomnia and fatigue but also leptin resistance. Overeating and eating too close to bedtime fall into the same category. Who hasn't tossed, turned, and had bad dreams from that late-night pizza, Buffalo wings, or birthday cake? Reducing any interference with a good night's rest helps to reset your leptin receptors and assists in weight loss.

High triglycerides, cholesterol, and blood sugar
Recent studies at both Yale and the University of California have shown that both cholesterol and triglycerides are not produced from the fat we consume. They are the result of sugar and carb consumption, as are high levels of blood sugar. If you have been told your levels in any of these areas are high, it's very probable that they have also promoted leptin resistance.

According to Dr. Richard Herbold of New York's Capital

District Vitality Center, "High triglycerides have been shown to block leptin. Diets high in alcohol, sugars and carbohydrate-rich foods, such as breads, pasta, rice, and potatoes, raise triglycerides considerably. High triglycerides have been shown to block the ability of leptin to pass into the brain to tell it you're full." ["Are You Always Hungry? You Could Have Leptin Resistance". 11/5/2012. www.capitaldistrictvitalitycenter.com]

Unfortunately, insulin resistance is not the only problem faced by diabetics and pre-diabetics. Insulin resistance and leptin resistance walk hand in hand. The process goes like this: "The more you eat, the more insulin you make, and the more leptin you make ... When ... cells don't need any sugar, then insulin stimulates the production of triglycerides, which can become stored fat ... Unfortunately, as triglycerides elevate in your blood they get in the way of leptin getting into your brain. This keeps you eating more than you need to because you don't yet have a full signal, a problem called leptin resistance. This encourages even further insulin driven triglyceride formation" (Richards, Byron J. www.wellnessresources.com/health/articles/insulin_leptin and_blood_sugar_why_diabetic_medication_fails)

It's a vicious cycle, where hormones are working against each other instead of in harmony.

Allergies and Food Sensitivities
Many allergies and food sensitivities are ultimately linked to the inflammation caused by food additives and artificial sweeteners, which block leptin receptors and cause leptin resistance. However, food sensitivities can manifest as such a startling array of symptoms such that many people don't realize what's really happening. According to weightloss-dietfree.com, "People with food sensitivities exhibit a wide variety of symptoms including fatigue, digestive disorders (constipation, diarrhea, flatulence, heartburn, burping, bloating), water retention, food cravings, headaches and migraines, skin rashes and eczema, sinus infections, nasal congestion, ear throat infections, ADD, ADHD, tantrums, irritability, bed-wetting, asthma, constantly clearing throat,

muscle aches, and much more." (www.weightloss-dietfree.com/leptin-resistance-4.html retrieved 7/1/2015)

If you experience these types of symptoms after eating particular foods, or if you know that you have allergies, you may already be leptin resistant.

Reproductive Issues

Nature can 'switch off' reproductive ability if there's not enough energy being registered by the system to produce a viable offspring. "The primary source of energy stores in people by far is fat, as many unfortunately are all too aware of. The primary signal that indicates how much fat is stored is leptin, and it is also leptin that allows for reproduction, or not. It has long been known that women with very little body fat, such as marathon runners, stop ovulating. There is not enough leptin being produced to permit it", explains Dr. Ron Rosedale in his article "Leptin And Its Essential Role In Health, Disease, And Aging" (Internet shared .pdf, retrieved 7/2/2015).

In leptin resistance, there's plenty of leptin, too much leptin in fact, but *the body doesn't register its presence.* This produces the same end result as insufficient leptin. It can result in a number of different reproductive issues, not just for women. Low testosterone levels in men have recently been linked to leptin resistance.

In summary, there are many signs and symptoms of leptin resistance. Those of us who have been eating the typical high-carbohydrate diet and using pre-packaged 'convenience' foods are very likely to have at least some degree of leptin resistance already, and those who are overweight definitely do. Dietary changes and exercise are the keys to resetting your leptin sensitivity and getting your metabolism back on track to prevent long-term health issues.

Chapter IV: The Long-Term Effects of Leptin Resistance

It's long been known that obesity is a major contributing factor for many serious diseases, although no one knew why. Leptin provides the missing link. The discovery of leptin was originally viewed as the panacea for obesity; take a leptin pill and lose weight! Unfortunately, this idea soon had to be abandoned since it didn't work at all. Now we understand why. It's not a lack of leptin that causes weight gain; rather it's an overabundance of it, desensitizing the system and keeping your brain from 'reading' the leptin. Leptin resistance is a 'hot issue' in scientific research right now. If we can reduce obesity, we can reduce the risks of developing most major health problems and extend our good health well into old age.

It's important to address leptin resistance through diet and exercise, even before you develop a weight issue, if possible. So far, no pharmacological solutions have shown much promise. Oh yes, there are some web sites promoting various African and South American plants as the cure for leptin resistance. They all cite various pieces of scientific evidence. However, no major scientific studies have backed up their claims at this point in time. The 'studies' that they quote are all their own and have not been validated by any objective independent sources. Diet and exercise **can** reduce and reverse your leptin resistance, but you have to work at it.

"Studies have now shown that leptin, or more correctly the inability of the body to properly hear leptin's signals (in other words leptin resistance), plays a significant if not primary role in heart disease, obesity, diabetes, osteoporosis, autoimmune diseases, reproductive disorders, and perhaps the rate of aging itself. It helps to control the brain areas that regulate thyroid levels and the sympathetic nervous system which also has huge impacts on blood pressure, heart disease, diabetes, osteoporosis and aging." (Rosedale, Ron. "Leptin And Its Essential Role In Health, Disease, And Aging". Internet shared .pdf, retrieved 7/2/2015).

That's an amazing list, isn't it? It's like a laundry list of the degenerative age-related illnesses. Most of the problems stem from the interplay of the various hormones, and there are many researchers working to unravel this intricate puzzle. Because leptin stands at the helm of the ship, when it's not functioning correctly, nothing else will be for long either. Leptin resistance keeps the 'this body needs fuel' switch open all the time, resulting in the release (or non-release) of other hormones. The complex biochemistry that keeps us functioning as a finely-tuned machine starts to break down, and these hiccoughs and glitches in our body's workings end up producing seemingly unrelated problems, like reproductive disorders.

I'm not going to attempt to explain the complicated relationship between leptin resistance and all the above-mentioned illnesses. If you're of a scientific bent and truly interested in the 'why', you can look it up on the Internet and plough through the published research studies. They're interesting but also heavy going as reading material. There are, however, two broad areas that I will go into a little detail about here.

The first is the aspect of carrying excess weight. Extra pounds are not a cosmetic issue but a health issue. A study published in *The New England Journal of Medicine* in 2008 showed that as little as two inches of excess around the middle increased the risk of death for women by 13% and for men by 17%. Two inches! I've already talked about the obesity-insulin-leptin triangle that can cause or worsen diabetes, but that's not the only danger. According to Dr. Joseph Mercola, "At least 20 different diseases and conditions are directly attributable to being overweight. This societal problem has emerged in just the past four decades, in large part due to sorely misguided dietary guidelines." (www.articles.mercola.com/sites/articles/archive/2012/10/29/leptin-resistance.aspx)

One of those diseases is cancer. Being overweight causes cancerous tumors to grow more quickly, and as they grow they can metastasize to other locations in the body. The research of Mikhail Kolonin, published Oct. 15th, 2012, in *Cancer Research*, showed that the presence of cancer triggers 'white' fat cells to enter the bloodstream and travel to the site of the tumor. Once there, they provide both oxygen and nutrients to help the tumor grow more rapidly. This happens regardless of whatever treatment or diet the patient is following. In other words, cancer feeds off excess body fat, which explains the eventual wasting away of cancer patients. Losing the extra pounds can inhibit the growth of cancerous tumors, and controlling weight may help to prevent the disease from getting a toehold in your body in the first place.

The second area to explain, inflammation, is also the subject of a lot of scientific research at the moment. Quite a few diseases are currently being linked to excess inflammation. This is internal, sometimes cellular level, inflammation. Heart disease, stroke, diabetes, and even dementia and depression seem to be tied to inflammation, although the exact relationships are not yet clearly understood. (Scolaro, Laura, et al. "Leptin-Based Therapeutics"<<www.medscape.com/viewarticle/733348>>.Retrieved 7/1/2015.)

Not only is a high level of leptin very inflammatory by itself, but it also promotes the production of other pro-inflammatory substances in the body, particularly from fat cells. These have already been shown in several studies to speed the progression of heart disease and diabetes, and their relationship to other major diseases is being investigated.

Leptin, however, is not the only causative factor in producing inflammation in the human body. Other hormones, such as the stress hormone cortisol, contribute their share to the problem. One main factor, alluded to earlier by Dr. Joseph Mercola, is diet. There appear to be many substances in our food today that actively cause this internal inflammation, therefore producing the conditions to develop serious disease. Chemical additives, artificial colors, and artificial sweeteners rank particularly high on that list, as do fructose and the factory produced 'trans-fats'.

Many people suspect that genetically-modified plants, like many of the vegetable and fruits currently available, are also contributors to systemic inflammation. The non-toxic molds found in many foods, such as coffee and tea, add their degree of inflammation as well. These are all 'modern' problems, created by the rise of agri-business and the increasing use of pre-packaged foods with their 'hidden' ingredients, which have sharply risen in the past forty to fifty years. The strong advertising push for consumption of cold cereals and sweet beverages, such as soda pop and 'energy' drinks, has also contributed to the pollution of our bodies on a daily basis. Its effect on our health and longevity has been frightening.

The growing popularity of organic and 'heritage' foods, grass-fed beef, and free-range chickens and their eggs comes from people's desire to remove these suspect ingredients from the dinner table. People who have done so have reported relief from health issues ranging from sinus and allergy problems to fibromyalgia to irritable bowel syndrome. Unfortunately, at the present time these foodstuffs remain on the expensive side, outside the range of many family budgets. You can, however, reduce this type of systemic inflammation by reading labels to find the 'cleanest' products that you can. Avoiding the 'worst offenders' among the additives can go a long way in lowering overall inflammation in the body.

Of course, decreasing your leptin resistance will be a huge stride towards reducing low-grade systemic inflammation as well. As leptin receptors return to 'listening' to your leptin levels, hunger and cravings decrease, appetite becomes regulated, and hormone levels return to a healthy rate across the board. The pro-inflammatory hormones and chemicals are greatly reduced, allowing your system to heal and function normally.

As more research is completed, we will begin to better understand the intricate interweaving of diet, hormones, and health. For now, it's enough to know that there are several things you can do to reverse your leptin resistance and improve your health, both short and long term. Diet and exercise will set you back on the road to a long and healthy life.

Chapter V: Ready, Set, ... Reset!

The Leptin Resistance Reset is built around the following five basic rules:

1. Stop eating at least three hours before going to bed.
2. Eat only three meals a day, about 5-6 hours apart. No snacking.
3. Limit meal size and stop *before* you feel 'full'.
4. Have a breakfast (with lots of protein) within 30 minutes of getting up.
5. Limit carbohydrates and eliminate food additives.

Before we look at a 14-day meal plan, let's talk about the general strategy for eating to lower your leptin resistance and how to integrate it into your daily routine. You don't need to obsess over percentages or calories with this diet, but you do need to pay attention to some guidelines.

Each meal should contain between 400 and 600 calories. While you will be decreasing the amount of carbohydrate you eat, you'll also be increasing the amount of healthy fat you consume. This is a win-win for you because fats keep you feeling satisfied longer, and they are not stored as body fat like carbs are. Your goal is to have the optimal balance of macronutrients for ideal hormone functioning. That works out to be 40% fats, 30% proteins, and 30% carbohydrates.

Entering your meals into a calculator is the easiest way to track both calories and percentages, and there are a number of easy-to-use ones available for use on your computer or mobile device. Figure your protein needs by taking 50-60% of your *ideal* body weight. That's how many *grams* of protein you should eat daily. Build you other macronutrient figures around that.

Drink a lot of water and no-calorie drinks because thirst is often mistakenly 'read' as hunger. Many herbal teas are terrific as iced tea, but you need to be wary of the bottled varieties, which often contain added sweeteners and artificial ingredients. You also want to stay away from so-called 'energy drinks'. Eliminate sugar and artificial sweeteners for reasons already discussed. Use only Stevia to sweeten, and investigate the wide selection of flavored liquids available for sweetening everything from coffee to yogurt. [You can make terrific lemonade with just water, Stevia, and lemon juice.] Use real cream in your coffee or tea in place of artificial 'creamers', which are high in sugars and additives. Also eliminate anything containing soy since it has been proven to inhibit weight loss, and read food labels to avoid additives and 'hidden' ingredients.

Consider these changes and adjustments as a 'work in progress'. Every step towards these goals is a stride towards fat loss and better health, both short-term and long. Be patient with yourself, don't expect perfection, and take it as slowly as you need. If you experience hunger and cravings, it's a signal that your body is still not listening to your leptin! You may want to consider doing a 3-day 'quick start' by having nothing but protein shakes and smoothies for three days and then starting the meal plan over again. Personally, I find it easier to fight hunger and cravings by drinking *lots* of water and getting away from food by taking the dog for a walk. I also check my fat and protein consumption to make sure I'm getting enough. If your intake of fats is high, they will keep you feeling full and help to fight cravings.

Let's talk about shopping for some of those items that turn up regularly in the meal plan. Bread products of any sort (pita, wraps, etc.) should be whole-grain and additive-free, so read labels. Oatmeal is a tremendous food, especially for breakfast, because it's filling and provides protein along with many other nutrients. It's important, however, to buy 'real' oatmeal, not the overly processed 'instant', which contains sugar among other things. Regular rolled oats are fine, as are steel-cut (or Irish). Both cook quickly and easily on the stovetop, in the microwave, or in the slow cooker. Choose full-fat or 2% dairy products because you need to increase your intake of fats. Full-fat dairy also appears to block the absorption of other less healthy fats in food, according to a 2014 Canadian study. Be very careful buying yogurt and really read those labels! Yogurt very often has added sugar or artificial sweeteners. Buy plain yogurt and sweeten it yourself with fresh fruit or Stevia.

Finally, most smoothies call for added protein powder, and this is an area that can be tricky to navigate. The protein can be taken from many different sources, and any particular brand may (or may not) contain sugar and other additives. Look for a product without unnecessary additives. *Whey protein* is the most 'complete', meaning it contains all the essential amino acids your own body doesn't produce. It's also absorbed the most quickly and is great for building and maintaining muscles, which burn more calories than fat. *Casein protein* is absorbed more slowly by your body, but it also keeps you feeling 'full' longer, so it's very good for smoothies or added to morning oatmeal for a protein boost.

Many people combine these two types of supplemental protein powders, using a scoop of each, to maximize the benefits of a breakfast or lunch smoothie. *Prevention* magazine highly recommends the following three protein powders: Source Organic Grass-Fed Whey Protein Concentrate, Now Foods Whey Isolate, and Naked Casein. (Ecklecamp, Stephanie. "The Six Healthiest Protein Powders for Your Smoothie". *Prevention*. 1/14/2015. http://www.prevention.com))

Do your homework thoroughly before making your choice, and seek assistance from a sales associate. Also, although a big jar may seem pretty expensive, you need to remember that it will only be used a scoop or two at a time. You'll quickly find yourself tossing it into all sorts of things because protein keeps hunger at bay!

The meal plan that follows is meant to be a guide, not gospel. Change it around to suit your life, your schedule, and your tastes. Also, add proteins and adjust the portion size to meet your individual needs. You can always add more non-starch veggies to just about any meal. Planning ahead, and cooking ahead, will make it easier to prepare all of these meals, and a blender and a slow cooker will simplify things a lot. There are also planned leftovers to save you some time.

The recipes for the dishes marked will be found in the next chapter.

Two-Week Meal Plan

Day 1:
- Breakfast: 2 eggs, any style, 4 slices bacon, optional whole-grain toast
- Lunch: Quinoa Salad
- Dinner: Greek Stuffed Chicken

Day 2:
- Breakfast: Overnight Oatmeal
- Lunch: leftover Greek Stuffed Chicken in a pita
- Dinner: Steak Burrito

Day 3:
- Breakfast: Super Coffee Smoothie
- Lunch: Crab Salad
- Dinner: Cauli Fried Rice

Day 4:
- Breakfast: Steak (4 oz.) and 2 eggs
- Lunch: Stuffed Avocado
- Dinner: Coconut Crusted Chicken with Roasted Vegetables

Day 5:
- Breakfast: Crockpot Oatmeal
- Lunch: Greek Salad
- Dinner: Veggie Lasagna

Day 6:
- Breakfast: Breakfast Pudding
- Lunch: Hamburger Soup and a green salad
- Dinner: Shrimp Lo Mein

Day 7:
- Breakfast: Mini Frittatas
- Lunch: Egg Salad
- Dinner: Coffee Braised Beef

Day 8:
- Breakfast: Salmon Muffins
- Lunch: Creamy Broccoli Soup with green salad
- Dinner: Chicken in a Pot

Day 9:
- Breakfast: Overnight Oatmeal
- Lunch: leftover Coffee Braised Beef in pita or salad
- Dinner: Dinner Salad with leftover Salmon Muffins

Day 10:
- Breakfast: Lemon Snap Smoothie
- Lunch: Quinoa Salad with Chicken
- Dinner: Stuffed Peppers

Day 11:
- Breakfast: 2 eggs and 4 slices bacon
- Lunch: Creamy Broccoli Soup with green salad & leftover Mini Frittatas
- Dinner: Poached Fish with Roasted Veggies

Day 12:
- Breakfast: Crockpot Oatmeal
- Lunch: leftover Poached Fish in tacos or wraps
- Dinner: Barbacoa Meatballs with Guacamole

Day 13:
- Breakfast: Iced Mega-Coffee
- Lunch: Salad with leftover Meatballs
- Dinner: African Chicken Stew

Day 14:
- Breakfast: 2 poached eggs on whole-grain toast with sausage
- Lunch: Chicken Salad
- Dinner: Steak Burrito

Chapter VI: Leptin-Friendly Recipes

Enjoy making and eating the following recipes, and make substitutions and adjust serving size to better suit your individual tastes and nutritional needs. Most slow cooker recipes can also be done on the stovetop in a large stockpot, and don't forget to cook and freeze extras for quick easy meals later on.

Quinoa Salad

This salad makes a great introduction to the South American grain quinoa, which is one of the few grains high in protein. It's both filling and delicious, and it also makes a healthy stand-in for rice or potatoes in many dishes. [3 servings]

Ingredients:
- ½ cup quinoa
- 8 oz. fresh mozzarella, cut bite-sized
- cherry or grape tomatoes, halved
- chopped fresh basil
- 2 T olive oil
- salt & pepper to taste

Preparation:
1. In a medium saucepan, boil 1 cup of water. Add the quinoa, reduce heat to simmer, and cook until all the water is absorbed, about 15 minutes. Cool the quinoa in the fridge.
2. Mix the cooled quinoa with the tomatoes and cheese, then add the basil. Mix well, drizzle with olive oil, and add salt and pepper.
3. Serve either at room temperature or chilled.

Nutrition Information per serving: 415 calories, 24.6 g fat, 24.6 g carbohydrates (2.5 g fiber), 25.9 g protein

Greek Stuffed Chicken

You can make fantastic stuffed chicken breasts in the slow cooker, and they'll stay moist and delicious. Once you try these Greek stuffed breasts, you'll go crazy creating your own. This recipe is low in fat, so pair it with a high-fat side dish or drizzle some butter onto those veggies. [6 servings]

Ingredients:
- 6 6-8 oz. boneless skinless chicken breasts
- 3 cups finely chopped spinach
- 2 roasted red peppers, chopped
- 1/4 cup sliced black olives
- 1 cup artichoke hearts, chopped
- 4 oz. feta cheese
- 1 tbsp. oregano, chopped
- 1 tsp. garlic powder
- 1.5 cups chicken broth
- Salt and pepper

Preparation:
1. In a bowl, combine the spinach, red peppers, olives, artichoke hearts, feta, oregano, and garlic powder. Mix well.
2. Season the chicken breasts with salt and pepper. Make a deep cut from the side into the center of the chicken breast, but don't cut all the way through. This makes the pocket.
3. Fill the pocket with the spinach mixture and place them in the slow cooker on their sides, with the pockets facing up.
4. Pour the chicken broth into the crock-pot, and then cover and cook on low for about 4 hours.

Nutrition Information per serving: 210 calories, 6.7 g fat, 4.3 g carbohydrates (0.5 g fiber), 34.1 g protein

Overnight Oatmeal

This is an effortless 'no cook' way to make oatmeal --- in your refrigerator! It's affordable and very healthy with protein, whole grain, and fresh fruit. Create your own combinations using frozen fruit as well. [2 servings]

Ingredients:
- 1-1/2 cups regular rolled oats
- 1 cup unsweetened almond milk or coconut milk
- 1 tsp lemon zest
- 3 scoops protein powder
- ½ tsp vanilla extract
- ¼ cup chopped pecans, walnuts, or almonds
- fresh or frozen raspberries

Preparation:
1. Combine oats, milk, lemon zest, and vanilla in a bowl. Cover and refrigerate overnight.
2. To serve, divide into portions and heat in microwave (if you want it warmed). Top with nuts and fruit, and thin with a little more milk as needed.

Nutrition Information per serving: 435 calories, 8.5 g fat, 25 g carbohydrates (6.7 g fiber), 42 g protein

Steak Burrito

Marinate the steak all day in the fridge for cooking in the evening. This is a satisfying end to the day when paired with a fresh green salad. [4 servings]

Ingredients:
- ½ cup salsa
- ½ cup water
- ¼ cup uncooked brown rice
- 1 15-oz. can black beans (drained)
- 12 oz. strip steak, trimmed and sliced diagonally and thinly
- 1 T coconut or olive oil
- 4 whole-wheat tortillas
- ½ cup shredded cheddar cheese
- ¼ cup guacamole or sliced avocado
- 2 T fresh cilantro, chopped
- Marinade: blend until smooth 2 jalapenos (seeded and diced), ¼ cup cumin seeds, ¾ cup olive oil, 1 bunch cilantro stems and leaves, 1 tsp salt, 1 T black pepper, 1 clove garlic (crushed), ½ cup lime juice

Preparation:
1. Marinate the steak slices overnight or all day in the refrigerator.
2. Cook the rice following the directions on the package. With 10 minutes left of cooking time, add the salsa and the extra ½ cup water. Simmer for 5 minutes and then stir in the beans. Simmer uncovered until rice is tender and the liquid is absorbed.
3. Heat a large skillet over medium-high heat and melt the oil. Cook the steak strips about 3-5 minutes, turning and stirring, until meat is cooked through.
4. Divide all the ingredients onto the tortillas. Fold in the sides and roll up.

Nutrition Information per serving: 471 calories, 16 g fat, 48 g carbohydrates, 31 g protein

Super Coffee Smoothie

A big mug of enhanced coffee is a great start to many a morning! You can also try this with plain yogurt and a few drops of flavored Stevia to change things up. It may just become your 'go-to' breakfast! [1 serving]

Ingredients:
- 2 scoops protein powder
- 10-12 oz. coffee (room temperature or cold)
- 8 oz. vanilla yogurt
- 3-5 ice cubes

Preparation:
1. Add all ingredients to the blend and mix until smooth.

Nutrition Information per serving: 161 calories, 2.8 g fat, 16 g carbohydrates, 45 g protein

Crab Salad

Crab is always rich and filling, and this recipe rolls it together with green beans and a tart apple for crunch. This makes a great dinner as well, or make extra for some leftovers for another lunch. [2 servings]

Ingredients:
- 1-1/2 cups frozen green beans
- 2 T coarse sea salt
- 1 cup Greek yogurt
- 1 T Dijon mustard
- 1/4 tsp salt
- 4 T fresh chives, minced
- 1 Granny Smith apple, peeled, cored, and cubed
- 1 ripe avocado, peeled, pitted, and cubed
- 8 oz. cooked lump crabmeat (about 1 cup)

Preparation:
1. Bring a large pot of water to a rolling boil. Put beans into a colander along with coarse salt. Immerse in the boiling water for 3-4 minutes. Remove from water and rinse with cold water. Drain and pat dry.
2. Mix the mustard and salt into the yogurt in a large bowl. Add the beans, chives, avocado, and crab. Stir to mix well before serving.

Nutrition Information per serving: 220 calories, 9 g fat, 17 g carbohydrates, 20 g protein

Cauli Fried Rice

A lower carb version of your favorite fried rice, feel free to make your own additions and substitutions. Add some meat to this or pair it with a baked or broiled protein of choice. Cauliflower rice is lighter and more nutritious than rice, and you can 'rice' a lot of it ahead of time and keep it in the freezer for quick meals later on. [2 servings]

Ingredients:
- 1 head of cauliflower
- 3 eggs, whisked
- 1 lb. package frozen peas and carrots (or veggie mix of choice)
- 1 T tamari sauce or coconut aminos [soy sauce substitute]

Preparation:
1. Divide cauliflower into flowerets that will fit in a food processor. Pulse until you have small rice-sized bits.
2. In a large pot, melt some oil and cook the cauli rice over medium heat, stirring regularly to prevent burning.
3. Cook your frozen veggies for 5-10 minutes in boiling water, or in the microwave.
4. Heat oil over medium heat to cook the eggs. Stir the eggs to keep cooked pieces small. When they are pretty firm, add the cooked eggs to the cauli rice in the big pot.
5. Drain the veggies and add them to the cauli-egg mix in the big pot. Stir in tamari and salt to taste. Cook together for 3-4 minutes before serving.

Nutrition Information per serving: 280 calories, 7 g fat, 37 g carbohydrates (14 g fiber), 19 g protein

Stuffed Avocado

This sounds like a light lunch, but avocado is very rich in healthy fats. It will keep you full for quite a while! Add a couple of shrimp or a little chicken to bump up the protein. [1 serving]

Ingredients:
- 1 ripe avocado
- ¼-1/2 cup cottage cheese
- small tomato, diced
- wedge of lemon
- salt

Preparation:
1. Cut avocado in half and remove the pit.
2. Fill each half with cottage cheese.
3. Top each half with diced tomatoes and a sprinkle of salt. Spritz with lemon juice.

Nutrition Information per serving: 420 calories, 39 g fat, 19 g carbohydrates (14 g fiber), 5 g protein

Coconut-Crusted Chicken

You can also use shrimp for this recipe, and most white fish is good 'coconut-crusted' as well. It's delicious and simple to make.

Ingredients:
- Shredded unsweetened coconut flakes or powder
- Sea salt
- Fresh parsley
- Dried oregano
- 1 lb. chicken breast or thighs, cut into strips
- 2 eggs

Preparation:
1. Preheat oven to 325 degrees F.
2. Mix the coconut, salt, parsley, and oregano in one bowl. In another bowl, beat the eggs until well blended.
3. Dip the chicken into the egg and then roll in in the dry mix until coated. Bake until it starts to brown.

Nutrition Information per serving: 290 calories, 8.3 g fat, 0.2 g carbohydrates, 52 g protein

Roasted Veggies

This is a quick easy way to make veggies more interesting, especially for kids. Brussels sprouts, broccoli, and cauliflower are terrific done in the oven, and carrots and zucchini take on a 'French fry' type of appeal. Adjust cook time depending on your chosen vegetables and the size that you cut them.

Ingredients:
- Veggies of choice
- Olive oil
- Salt

Preparation:
1. Clean and cut veggies into bite-sized pieces.
2. Toss veggies in a little olive oil, and then spread on a baking sheet.
3. Sprinkle with salt and bake at 350 until tender, about 20-30 minutes.

Crockpot Oatmeal

Here is wonderful oatmeal you can start before bed and have ready for eating when you wake up. Although it's handy to make during the workweek, it's equally great for a lazy Saturday morning. Change the fruit or add nuts if you like, or try adding vanilla, cinnamon, pumpkin pie spice, or another flavor to your oatmeal. [4 servings]

Ingredients:
- 8 cups water
- 2 cups steel-cut oats
- 2 scoops protein powder
- 1/3 cup dried cranberries
- 1/3 cup dried apricots, chopped
- ¼ teaspoon salt, or to taste

Preparation:
Combine water, oats, dried cranberries, dried apricots, and salt in a 5 or 6-quart slow cooker. Turn heat to low. Cover and cook until oats are tender and porridge is creamy, 7 to 8 hours.

Nutrition Information per serving: 195 calories, 3 g fat, 34 g carbohydrates, 32 g protein

Greek Salad

A hearty salad with strong Mediterranean flavors, this will keep you going until dinnertime. This recipe uses chicken, but you can substitute any other protein easily, which can be a great way to use up bits and dabs of leftovers. [4 servings]

Ingredients:
- 1/3 cup red wine vinegar
- 2 T olive oil
- 1 T chopped fresh oregano (or 1 tsp dried)
- 1 tsp garlic powder
- 1/4 tsp salt
- 1/4 tsp freshly ground pepper
- 6 cups baby spinach
- 2 1/2 cups chopped cooked chicken
- 2 medium tomatoes, chopped
- 1 medium cucumber, peeled, seeded and chopped
- 1/2 cup finely chopped red onion
- 1/2 cup sliced ripe black olives
- 1/2 cup crumbled feta cheese

Preparation:
1. In a large bowl, whisk together the vinegar, herbs, and spices.
2. Add all remaining ingredients to the bowl. Toss well to coat with the dressing.

Nutrition Information per serving: 296 calories, 16 g fat, 7.5 g carbohydrates (2.2 g fiber), 32 g protein

Veggie Lasagna
Mushrooms give this vegetarian dish a rich meaty texture, and the zucchini keeps it light. Like many other lasagnas, it is almost better the next day. [4 servings]

Ingredients:
- 2 T. olive oil
- 2 cups mushrooms, sliced
- 6 cloves garlic, chopped
- 2 (14.5-oz.) cans no-salt-added diced tomatoes
- 1 tsp. teaspoon dried oregano
- 6 oz. baby spinach
- 8 oz. low-fat cottage cheese
- 2 medium zucchini, cut lengthwise into 1/4-inch slices
- 1/2 tsp. salt
- 9 no-boil lasagna noodles
- 2 cups shredded low-fat mozzarella cheese

Preparation:
1. Preheat oven to 350 degrees. Prepare an 8 x 12 glass baking pan by drizzling 1 T. of olive oil in the bottom.
2. Heat the remaining olive oil in a fry pan over medium heat. Cook the mushrooms for 5 minutes, and then add the half garlic, tomatoes, and ½ tsp. oregano. Let simmer for about 6 minutes.
3. Microwave the spinach with 2 T of water for about 2 minutes. Drain and squeeze to remain excess liquid. Mix with the cottage cheese and the remaining garlic and oregano.
4. Lay the zucchini slices across the width of the baking dish. Sprinkle with salt. Top with lasagna noodles.
5. Spread the spinach-cheese mixture in the pan as the next layer and top with more lasagna noodles.
6. Pour about half of the tomato sauce on top, spreading evenly. Cover with the remaining noodles. Top with the rest of the sauce, making sure all the noodles are

covered. Sprinkle with cheese.

7. Cover with foil and bake for about 35 minutes. Remove the foil and return to the oven until brown and bubbly on top.
8. Allow to sit a few minutes before trying to slice and serve.

Nutrition Information per serving: 295 calories, 12 g fat, 18 g carbohydrates (4.4 g fiber), 28.8 g protein

Breakfast Pudding

This is a big breakfast that's satisfyingly thick and super packed with protein. It makes a nice hearty lunch as well. You can use plain protein powder and blend in some fresh fruit and nuts for a little more taste variety. [1 serving]

Ingredients:
- 4 oz. cottage cheese
- 6 oz. Greek yogurt
- 1 scoop flavored protein powder

Preparation:
Toss in the blender and blend until smooth.

Nutrition Information per serving: 340 calories, 5.7 g fat, 4.4 g carbohydrates (0.5 g fiber), 60 g protein

Hamburger Soup

You can play around with the ingredients in this one to your heart's delight. Kale or spinach make a great addition. This soup freezes well and makes a great quick lunch. [6 servings]

Ingredients:
- 1 lb. carrots, grated
- 2 leeks (whites only), finely chopped
- 2 zucchini, cut into ribbons with a peeler
- fresh basil
- 2 stalks celery, chopped
- 2 lbs. ground beef, brought to room temperature
- 2 c bone broth
- 2 bay leaves

Preparation:
1. In a large soup pot, cook carrots, celery, and leeks on medium heat about 10 minutes. Add a handful of basil, the bay leaves, bone broth, zucchini ribbons, and ground beef (in pieces). Add enough water to cover.
2. Simmer on medium until the beef is done, about 20 minutes. Add a dash of olive oil and stir it in, then add salt to taste. Pull out the bay leaves before serving.

Nutrition Information per serving: 340 calories, 9.6 g fat, 14 g carbohydrates (3.2 g fiber), 48 g protein

Shrimp Lo Mein

This is a simple one-pan lo mein that uses parsnips instead of regular noodles. This raises the nutrition, keeps the flavor, and tastes great! It also makes a great introduction to using veggie noodles instead of pasta in other recipes. [4+ servings]

Ingredients:
- 1 lb. parsnips
- 2 cups green beans, chopped (fresh or frozen)
- 1 carrot, chopped
- 1 onion, thin sliced
- 1 lb. pre-cooked shrimp (fresh or frozen)
- 4 T coconut oil
- 1 tsp garlic powder
- ½ tsp pepper
- 1 tsp salt
- 2 T. tamari or coconut aminos
- 2 T fish sauce or oyster sauce

Preparation:
1. Use a spiral slicer or a peeler to make long thin strips of parsnip for the 'noodles'.
2. Melt the coconut oil in a large pan or wok. Add the carrot and sauté for 2 minutes.
3. Add the onion and green beans and sauté 2 more minutes.
4. Add the parsnip 'noodles' and cook on medium heat for 6-8 minutes, until all veggies are getting soft.
5. Add all the seasonings and stir well. [If the shrimp are still frozen, add them now and cover the pan. Steam for about 2 minutes.] If shrimp are thawed, cook veggies with seasonings for about 2 minutes before adding the shrimp. Cook until shrimp are hot through and veggies are tender.

Nutrition Information per serving: 383 calories, 16 g fat, 32 g carbohydrates (9 g fiber), 30.2 g protein

Mini Frittatas

These are quick to make and the recipe easily doubles. Make several batches and freeze them for quick breakfasts or lunches. They always enhance eating a green salad meal! [3 servings]

Ingredients:
- 8 large eggs
- 2 cups chopped veggies or meat
- 2 scoops unflavored protein powder
- 2 T fresh herbs of choice
- pinch of salt and pepper

Preparation:
1. Preheat oven to 375 degrees. Lightly grease a muffin pan.
2. In a large bowl, whisk eggs until frothy. Add salt and pepper.
3. Stir in the veggies and herbs. Pour into the cups of the muffin pan.
4. Bake for about 10 minutes, until lightly browned and a toothpick in the middle comes out clean. They'll really puff up in the oven and will collapse back down.
5. Let cool slightly before removing from pan and serving.

Nutrition Information per serving: 278 calories, 13 g fat, 11 g carbohydrates (1.8 g fiber), 30.2 g protein

Egg Salad

Whether you eat it alone, on a green salad, or in a pita, this egg salad is a step beyond. Spicy with cayenne and ultra rich with avocado, this will definitely fill you up! [2 servings]

Ingredients:
- 8 large hardboiled eggs, chopped
- 1/2 cup mayonnaise
- 1/2 cup salsa
- 1/2 cup onion, finely chopped
- 1/2 cup celery, finely chopped
- 1 large avocado
- 2 tablespoons lime juice
- salt and pepper, to taste
- cayenne pepper, to taste

Preparation:
1. Halve and pit the avocado. Scoop the meat into a large bowl, then add the lime juice, and mash.
2. Add in the mayo, salsa, onion, and celery and mix well.
3. Fold the eggs into the mixture, and season with salt, pepper, and cayenne.
4. Refrigerate for 30+ minutes to let the flavors blend nicely.

Nutrition Information per serving: 377 calories, 29 g fat, 15.9 g carbohydrates (4.4 g fiber), 15 g protein

Coffee Braised Beef

This recipe is both spicy and smoky, with a unique flavor from the coffee. Despite its long ingredient list, this is easy to prepare in a slow cooker. It's great served as a classic roast with mashed cauliflower. If there's any leftover, shred the meat for salads or wraps. [6-8 servings]

Ingredients:
- 2.5-3 lb. chuck roast
- 1 large red onion, sliced thickly
- 4 cloves garlic, minced or pressed
- 2 tsp. cocoa powder
- 3 Tbsp. ancho chili powder
- 1 tsp. oregano
- 1/8 tsp. cinnamon
- 1 tsp. cumin
- ½ tsp. chipotle powder
- ½ tsp. salt
- ¾ c. strong coffee
- 1 Tbsp. balsamic vinegar

Preparation:
1. First you'll make a spice rub by combining all the ingredients EXCEPT the beef, onion, coffee, and vinegar. Mix them well and then rub it into the meat, covering all sides.
2. Next, put the onion in the bottom of the crockpot. The meat goes on top of the onion. Finally, add the vinegar to the coffee, stir and pour it over the roast. Cook covered for 6-8 hours on low.

Nutrition Information per serving: 300 calories, 15 g fat, 2 g carbohydrates (1 g fiber), 41 g protein

Salmon Muffins

These little fish loaves are tasty, very portable, and easy to heat in the microwave for a quick lunch. They use almond flour, which you can find in the organic baking section in many large supermarkets. Double or triple the recipe and freeze the extras after baking. [3 servings]

Ingredients:
- 1 lb. salmon filets, skin removed [or equivalent of canned salmon]
- 1 stalk celery, chopped
- ½ onion, chopped
- 1 egg
- 1 4-oz. can diced green chilies
- ¼ cup almond flour
- 1 tsp. garlic powder
- 1 tsp. chipotle chili powder
- 1/2 T parsley
- Salt and pepper to taste

Preparation:
1. Grease the cups on a muffin pan and preheat oven to 350 degrees.
2. Put all the ingredients in a food processor and blend until well mixed.
3. Place a ¼ cup of mixture into each muffin cup, and bake for 30-35 minutes until they are just beginning to brown on the edges.

Nutrition Information per serving: 254 calories, 12 g fat, 4.8 g carbohydrates (0.6 g fiber), 32 g protein

Creamy Broccoli Soup

This makes lots, so freeze the extra in serving-sized containers for quick lunches or dinners. Try some shredded cheddar on top, and add some chicken to your salad to raise the protein content.

Ingredients:
- 6-8 cups broccoli florets
- 3-4 shallots, minced
- 1 carrot, sliced
- 4 c bone broth or veggie broth
- ½ cup butter
- Sea salt to taste

Preparation:
1. Put a dab of butter into a large stockpot and lightly sauté the shallots and carrot.
2. Add the broccoli and cook until it's bright green.
3. Pour in the broth and continue to cook until broccoli is tender.
4. Add the remaining butter and blend (a hand blender works well) until desired consistency. Season with sea salt and serve hot.

Nutrition Information per serving: 317 calories, 25 g fat, 16.2 g carbohydrates (5.1 g fiber), 11 g protein

Chicken in a Pot

This is a very versatile crockpot recipe that can make either a meal or the foundation for some great chicken soup. It's easy to add in other cut-up vegetables to expand this into a stew, and the cooking liquid also makes a good homemade chicken broth. [6 servings]

Ingredients
- 2 carrots, sliced
- 2 onions, sliced
- 2 stalks celery, cut into 1-inch pieces
- 3 lb. chicken, whole or cut up
- 2 tsp. salt
- ½ tsp. coarse black pepper
- 1 tsp. dried basil
- ½ c. water, chicken broth, or dry white wine

Preparation:
1. Mix your vegetables and put them in the bottom of the crock.
2. Add the chicken on top of them. Sprinkle with the seasonings and pour in your choice of liquid.
3. Cover and cook. On High, this cooks for 3 ½ -5 hours (add an extra ½ cup of liquid), but it can go for 8-10 hours on low.

Nutrition Information per serving: 150 calories, 3.3 g fat, 5.8 g carbohydrates (1.8 g fiber), 23 g protein

Lemon Snap Smoothie

This is a cool refreshing way to start your day with lots of fruit. The spinach gives it a real nutrient boost. [1 serving]

Ingredients:
- 1 orange, peeled
- ½ banana, peeled
- ½-inch thick slice of pineapple (with core)
- 1 large handful of fresh spinach
- 1 thin lemon slice with peel
- 1-1/2 cups of ice
- 1 scoop protein powder

Preparation:
Toss all ingredients in a blender and blend until smooth.

Nutrition Information per serving: 355 calories, 2.7 g fat, 62 g carbohydrates (10 g fiber), 27 g protein

Stuffed Peppers

Another classic meal made easy in the crockpot, but you can oven cook these as well. The slow cooking keeps these really moist, however, and they're quick to put together with no pre-cooking needed. [4 servings]

Ingredients:
- 4 bell peppers
- 1 lb. ground meat
- ½ head cauliflower
- 1 onion, diced
- 1 carrot, diced
- 4 garlic cloves, minced
- 6 oz. can tomato paste
- 1/4 c. Italian seasoning blend
- ¼ c. beef stock
- salt and pepper to taste

Preparation:
1. Neatly slice the tops off of your peppers, keeping them in one piece, and set aside. Clean the seeds out of the peppers.
2. Pulse your cauliflower, onion, carrot, and garlic in a food processor to get them as small as possible, or hand dice really tiny.
3. Mix the veggies with the meat, tomato paste, seasonings, and salt and pepper in a large bowl.
4. Once it's combined well, spoon the mixture into the bottoms of your peppers, filling them just to the top.
5. Put the filled peppers into the slow cooker and put the tops back on. Add the stock into the bottom of the crockpot, cover, and cook for 6-8 hours.

Nutrition Information per serving: 451 calories, 30 g fat, 23.2 g carbohydrates (6.7 g fiber), 24.2 g protein

Poached Fish

Simple poached fish is always a hit, and it gives you great leftovers for salads. The alcohol in the wine cooks off completely, but you can replace it with water if you'd like. You may substitute any fatty fish for the salmon. [4 servings]

Ingredients:
- 1 to 1 ½ pounds salmon fillets, pin bones removed
- sea salt
- ½ c dry white wine
- ½ c water
- 1 shallot, peeled and sliced
- several sprigs of fresh dill
- a sprig of fresh parsley

Preparation:
1. Put all ingredients except the salmon in a large pan. Bring to a simmer over medium heat.
2. Season the salmon fillets with a little salt. Place them skin-side down in the simmering liquid in the pan.
3. Cover and cook about 8 minutes, depending on the thickness of the fillets.

Nutrition Information per serving: 324 calories, 14 g fat, 0.8 g carbohydrates, 44 g protein

Barbacoa Meatballs with Guacamole

Quick and easy to make with all the healthy fat and richness of avocado --- who could ask for more? Save some for lunch tomorrow! [6 servings]

Ingredients:
- 2 lbs 80/20 ground beef
- 2 tsp granulated garlic
- 2 tsp ground cumin
- 2 tsp smoked paprika
- 2 tsp dried oregano
- salt to taste
- 1 tsp ground coriander
- 1/4 tsp cayenne pepper
- 1/4 tsp ground cinnamon
- zest from 1 lime

Guacamole: 2 ripe avocados, juice from 1 lime

Preparation:
1. Preheat oven to 400 degrees.
2. Combine all ingredients (except guacamole) in a large bowl and mix thoroughly.
3. Use a small ice cream scoop to portion out the meatballs or roll them by hand. Place them in a 13 X 9 baking dish and cook for 20-25 minutes.
4. Halve and pit the avocados. Scoop the meat into a bowl and mash well with the lime juice.
5. Serve meatballs on a platter surrounded by the guacamole for dipping.

Nutrition Information per serving: 418 calories, 22.5 g fat, 5.8 g carbohydrates 4.5 g fiber), 47.1 g protein

Iced Mega-Coffee

This is a yummy mocha start to your day. Add some yogurt to add more protein and calcium. [1 serving]

Ingredients:
- 2 scoops protein powder
- 8-10 oz. cold coffee
- 8 oz. chocolate/dark chocolate almond milk
- 4-5 ice cubes

Preparation:
1. Blend protein powder, coffee, and almond milk in a blender.
2. Pour over ice to serve.

Nutrition Information per serving: 330 calories, 6.2 g fat, 24 g carbohydrates (1 g fiber), 45.3 g protein

African Chicken Stew

Sweet potatoes, peanut butter, and spices give this chicken stew its traditional African flair. It's simple to prepare in the slow cooker, and it will add a whole new view of chicken to your meal planning. You can do the pre-cooking in the evening, store it in the refrigerator overnight, and pop it quickly into crockpot in the morning for all-day cooking.

Ingredients:
- 1 tsp. coconut oil
- ¼ tsp. sea salt
- 1 ¼ lbs. boneless chicken thighs, quartered
- ¼ cup peanut butter
- ¼ cup water
- ½ tsp garlic powder
- 10 oz. diced tomatoes and green chilies (undrained)
- 2 medium sweet potatoes, peeled and cut into 1 ½ inch pieces
- 2 cups bell pepper and onion strips

Preparation:
1. Salt the chicken thighs. In a large fry pan over medium-high heat, brown the chicken in the coconut oil.
2. Stir in the peanut butter, water, garlic powder, and the tomatoes/chilies, including the liquid from the can. Cook until blended and it coats the chicken.
3. Put the sweet potatoes, bell pepper, and onion in the bottom of the slow cooker. Add the chicken mixture on top.
4. Cover and cook on low for 7-9 hours until vegetable are tender.
5. Stir to mix before serving.

Nutrition Information per serving: 264 calories, 6.2 g fat, 15 g carbohydrates, 21 g protein

Chicken Salad

The cranberries not only add a surprise flavor to this chicken salad, but they also supply some great anti-oxidants. This is really quick to make and easy to take along to work. Serve with some pieces of toasted whole-wheat pita to boost the crunch factor. [4-6 servings]

Ingredients:
- 4 cups (about 2 lbs.) cubed cooked chicken
- 1 stalk of celery, diced
- 2 T finely chopped shallot
- 1 cup dried cranberries
- 2/3 cup olive-oil mayonnaise
- 3 T tarragon vinegar or white wine vinegar
- 2 T finely chopped fresh tarragon or basil
- 1/2 tsp salt
- 1/2 tsp black pepper
- chopped Romaine lettuce

Preparation:
1. Combine chicken, celery, shallot, and cranberries in a large bowl.
2. In a separate bowl, mix the mayo, vinegar, herbs, salt, and pepper. Blend well.
3. Add the mayo mix to the chicken mix. Stir to combine well.
4. Serve over Romaine lettuce.

Nutrition Information per serving: 378 calories, 14 g fat, 5.3 g carbohydrates (1.0 fiber), 52.8 g protein

Conclusion: Maintaining Your Success

Once you have your leptin receptors back in working order, you'll see your metabolism begin to regulate both your appetite and your weight properly. You'll feel better, sleep better, and improve your odds of living a long happy life.

It's important to remember, however, to avoid those things that will mess with your leptin and sabotage your success. Let me summarize them here for you:

- Keep meals in proportion, don't overeat, and don't snack.
- Avoid artificial sweeteners, hidden ingredients, and food additives.
- Keep carbohydrate intake low, and avoid sugars and starches.
- Start each day with a protein breakfast.
- Exercise mildly but regularly.
- Get enough sleep.
- Drink lots of water and other non-sweetened beverages.

If you suspect a return of your leptin resistance, jump right on it. It's easier (and quicker) to correct a small problem than a big one!

If you have been leptin resistant for a long time, don't expect your whole system to reset in just a few days. Give your body time to recover, and follow the guidelines given in this book as best you can. Every step forward leads to better health, better body weight, and improved overall well being. That's your end goal. It's time to start the journey right now and become all that you were meant to be. You **can** take control of your hormones and your life... and you **can** beat leptin resistance! RESET!

Made in the USA
Monee, IL
10 October 2022